Amal Samet

Epistaxis

Amal Samet

Epistaxis

PEC, severity and recurrence

ScienciaScripts

Imprint
Any brand names and product names mentioned in this book are subject to trademark, brand or patent protection and are trademarks or registered trademarks of their respective holders. The use of brand names, product names, common names, trade names, product descriptions etc. even without a particular marking in this work is in no way to be construed to mean that such names may be regarded as unrestricted in respect of trademark and brand protection legislation and could thus be used by anyone.

Cover image: www.ingimage.com

This book is a translation from the original published under ISBN 978-620-6-73020-0.

Publisher:
Sciencia Scripts
is a trademark of
Dodo Books Indian Ocean Ltd. and OmniScriptum S.R.L publishing group

120 High Road, East Finchley, London, N2 9ED, United Kingdom
Str. Armeneasca 28/1, office 1, Chisinau MD-2012, Republic of Moldova, Europe
Managing Directors: Ieva Konstantinova, Victoria Ursu
info@omniscriptum.com

Printed at: see last page
ISBN: 978-620-8-62382-1

PLAN

INTRODUCTION

Epistaxis is one of the most common ear, nose and throat (ENT) emergencies. It accounts for 33% of emergency ENT consultations and 24.57% of emergency hospitalisations [1, 2]. Their clinical presentation varies greatly, ranging from small intermittent bleeds that can be managed by the patient themselves at home, to more serious forms requiring medical attention and regularly pushing patients to the emergency department. Epistaxis can be serious because of its abundance or repetition. Several factors can influence the severity of epistaxis, including the patient's condition, the aetiology and the nature of the management [3, 4]. The clinician has an important role to play in identifying "dangerous" forms of initial or secondary epistaxis and initiating early, comprehensive and effective management in order to improve the prognosis.

1- EPIDEMIOLOGY

1-1- Age

Epistaxis is a common problem that can affect people of any age and the incidence and impact of epistaxis varies with age [5].

In the study by Ari et al, epistaxis was more common in the elderly due to age-related changes in the nasal mucosa and blood vessels.[6] In the Nepal study, the prevalence of epistaxis varied with age. The majority patients with epistaxis were in the 46-65 age group, followed by the >65 age group.[7]

However Li et al reported that the number of hospital visits for epistaxis was lowest in patients over 70 years of age and that patients under 40 years of age had a higher incidence rate of epistaxis [8]. In another study, the age distribution of patients over a 14-year period revealed that the number of cases of epistaxis was higher in younger patients than in older patients [9]. In this study, in which patients were included regardless age, annual incidence epistaxis was highest in the under-18 group (N=19580(41.99%)) and lowest patients aged over 70 (N=2675(5.74%)). In a paediatric population, according to a study by ElAlfy et al, mean age 7.89 ± 3.89 years. They also found that the incidence of epistaxis decreased after puberty and was rare in children under 2 years of age[10].

1-2- Gender

The prevalence of epistaxis by gender varies between studies. In the paediatric population, the sex distribution in the study showed an almost equal frequency ,with 53 female patients and 47 patients .[10] Li et al found a predominance of males in the series; this predominance was essentially in spontaneous epistaxis [8,11]. This male predominance is not constant since Ari et al found that the occurrence of epistaxis was more frequent in women during the period of the SARS-CoV-II pandemic[6].

1-3-Season

The influence of the season on the onset of epistaxis has been noted, but studies of the association between epistaxis and climatic events have produced inconsistent results.In a study conducted in the United States, the author revealed that epistaxis occurred more often in autumn and winter, when temperatures are lower [1, 12].

Tabassom et al found that epistaxis occurs more frequently in older patients and during colder months [13]. However, for patients under the age of 18, Elalfy found that there were significantly more patients with epistaxis in the warmer months of the year and fewer in the spring, which may be attributed to seasonal variations [10]. In addition, a Turkish study found that the occurrence of epistaxis was positively related to mean temperature. [14]

In a Chinese study, the authors indicate that non-septal haemorrhage is linked to the autumn and winter seasons. In addition, they mention that male sex and increased LDL were high risk factors for non-septal haemorrhage in winter and spring. There therefore appears to be a seasonal influence in the occurrence of non-septal haemorrhage, with a higher prevalence during the coldest months of the year. However, the authors do not provide information on the seasonal variation in septal haemorrhage [8].

1-4-History

We found that hypertension and diabetes were the most common comorbidities in patients with epistaxis in line with Li et al who demonstrated that hypertension, diabetes and dyslipidaemia were common in patients with non-septal haemorrhage[8]. Elalfy et al found that 17% of the paediatric population had co-morbidities. These comorbidities were local, such as allergic rhinitis and chronic sinusitis, and systemic, mainly diabetes mellitus and gastrointestinal disease [10].Althaus et al found that the prevalence of these comorbidities varied according to the specialty of the doctor consulted. In fact, arterial hypertension and atrial fibrillation/flutter were the most common comorbidities in patients consulting a general practitioner than in those consulting an ENT specialist. In addition, the study revealed that antithrombotic treatment was recorded in 18.5% of cases seen by GPs and in 16.7% of cases seen by ENT specialists[11].

It has been found that comorbidities are correlated with nasal epitaxy. In a study analysing the cytology of nasal scrapings, it was observed that the cytological picture of the nasal mucosa coincided with the diagnosis of various diseases, including allergic and non-allergic rhinitis[15].

Epistaxis is associated in some authors with several respiratory comorbidities such as allergic rhinitis and chronic sinusitis [16]. In another study, Cingoz et al found that chronic obstructive pulmonary disease is a respiratory comorbidity that can have extra-pulmonary effects, including epistaxis [17].

It has also been reported that emergency department visits for epistaxis increase with age, and that patients over 65 are more likely to present to the emergency department with epistaxis. However, the results of this studies suggest that the prevalence of epistaxis may be higher in younger people than in those over 70 if the effect hypertension is excluded [8].

1-5- Habits

is well known that smoking can have negative effects on the respiratory system. Smoking can irritate the nasal passages and increase the risk of developing respiratory infections, which can potentially contribute to the development of epistaxis. In addition, smoking can alter blood coagulation and increase blood pressure, which can further increase the risk of nosebleeds. The relationship between smoking and epistaxis has been endorsed by several authors [11, 18, 19].In a case series, some authors found that varenicline, a stop-smoking drug, was associated with bleeding events, including epistaxis [20,21].Indirect markers of alcohol abuse have been found in patients with epistaxis, indicating that patients with epistaxis may have a history of alcohol abuse [22,23]. This increased incidence may be explained alcohol-induced platelet dysfunction [24].

In a Chinese study, Li et al found no significant correlation between alcohol consumption and epistaxis in patients over 40, whereas the effect of alcohol consumption was demonstrated in patients aged under 40. [8]

Other lifestyle habits that may contribute to the risk of epistaxis include :

- Stress: Stress can increase blood pressure and heart rate, which can put more pressure on the blood vessels in the nose.
- Dehydration: Dehydration can dry out the nasal mucosa, making it more fragile and prone to bleeding.
- Malnutrition: A diet rich in processed foods and low in fruit and vegetables can also increase the risk of epistaxis. Processed foods are often high in salt and fat, which can contribute to high blood pressure. Fruit and vegetables are a good source of vitamins and minerals such as vitamins C and K, which are important for blood clotting.

2- CAUSES

2-1- Local causes

2-1-1- Inflammatory and infectious

It is well known that any inflammatory process can cause epistaxis. In chronic sinusitis, this has been explained by the formation of highly vascularised granular tissue in the nasal cavity, potentially leading to recurrent epistaxis. The percentage of epistaxis of inflammatory origin varies from one study to another: in a retrospective study including 104 patients hospitalised for epistaxis, it was observed that 5.8% of cases were associated with chronic rhino sinusitis [25]. In contrast, Varshney et al found that 19.3% of epistaxis was of infectious etiology [26].

2-1-2- Trauma

Epistaxis secondary to craniofacial trauma varies in severity, ranging from the trivial in simple contusions and fractures of the bones proper of the nose to the serious in epistaxis secondary to arterial injury, particularly fractures passing through the carotid canal [27]. Injected CT scans of the facial mass provide an accurate assessment of the lesions. The traumatic origin of epistaxis has been observed in 12.7% to 30.8% of cases from one study to another [25, 28].

In cases post-traumatic epistaxis, of great abundance occurring after free time, a carotid-cavernous aneurysm should be suspected [29, 30].

In iatrogenic post-operative epistaxis, bleeding may occur immediately after an operation or during removal. Surgeries potentially at risk of bleeding include turbinectomy, meatotomy, ethmoidectomy, sphenoidectomy and rhinoseptoplasty.

In addition to external trauma, internal trauma can cause epistaxis of varying severity. These internal traumas may be simple scratching or by a foreign body, frequently observed in children or the mentally retarded, and sometimes leading to septal perforation [31].

2-1-3- Tumoral

The association of epistaxis with other rhino-logical signs (nasal obstruction, anosmia), ophthalmological signs (exophthalmos, diplopia, reduced visual acuity) and neurological signs (headache) should suggest the tumoral origin of the epistaxis, especially if the symptoms are unilateral [4].

In tumour forms, epistaxis may be secondary to direct vascular invasion or to the release of inflammatory mediators and cellular destruction products [32].

The incidence of tumour-induced epistaxis varies considerably in the literature, ranging from 1% to 18.2% [25, 26, 33, 34]. Malignant tumours such as squamous cell carcinoma, adenocarcinoma, melanoma, neuroblastoma of the nasal cavity and undifferentiated carcinoma of the nasopharynx (UCNT) have the highest incidence.Other than malignant tumours, certain benign tumours may be secondary to epistaxis, the most frequently described of which is the nasopharyngeal fibroma [4]: this is a hypervascularised tumour developed in the pterygo-palatine fossa, mainly affecting adolescent males, often developing at the age of puberty [35, 36]. In pregnant women, recurrent epistaxis secondary to an angiofibroma of the nasal septum may develop in the area of the vascular spot.

2-2- General causes

2-2-1- HTA

Hypertension, or high blood pressure, has been shown to be a common risk factor for epistaxis. Several studies have examined the relationship between hypertension and epistaxis. The prevalence of hypertension in patients epistaxis ranged from 24% to [37]. A systematic review of the literature found an association between hypertension and epistaxis [38]. Another study found that headache and epistaxis were the most common presenting signs of hypertensive emergencies [39].

Epistaxis can be secondary to unknown hypertension, with a high prevalence. In a study comparing two groups of patients without and with epistaxis in patients with unknown hypertension, Acar et al [40] found that 33.3% of patients with epistaxis were hypertensive compared with 11.7% of controls without epistaxis, the difference being significant (p=0.004).

Another retrospective study of 133 cases of essential epistaxis revealed higher systolic blood pressure values in patients with persistent bleeding (181.3 ± 26.9 vs 156.6 ± 26.1 mm Hg, $p < 0.0001$). These hypertensive patients also showed a higher prevalence of higher incidence of persistent epistaxis despite treatment (26% vs 8%, $p = 0.002$). Multivariate analysis identified systolic blood pressure as an independent factor associated with persistent bleeding (odds ratio 1.03; 95% confidence interval [1.01-1.06]; $p = 0.002$) [41].

In a systematic review of the literature involving 9 studies [42]the author affirmed the causal relationship between epistaxis and blood pressure level without taking into account the blood pressure value at the time of bleeding in order to eliminate the biases associated with stress and the white coat effect. It is important to note that although hypertension is a common risk factor for epistaxis, it is not always the direct cause. Other local and systemic factors may also contribute to the development of epistaxis [43].

2-2-2- **Haemostasis disorder**

Patients with haemostasis disorders or a disturbed coagulogram have several risk factors for epistaxis [13,44]. Furthermore, the use of drugs that alter haemostasis, such as anti-vitamin K, heparin, platelet aggregation inhibitors, direct thrombin inhibitors and direct factor Xa inhibitors, was also associated with an increased risk of epistaxis [45,46].

In statistics, epistaxis was secondary to the use of VKAs in 60,000 patients between 2006 and 2008 [47]. In a study of over 10,000 patients, Rainsbury et al found that the use antiplatelet agents increased the risk of epistaxis by 5 to 10 times [48].

The effect of antiplatelet agents may be increased by the use of non-steroidal anti-inflammatory drugs, thus increasing the risk epistaxis [49].

The risk epistaxis exists in patients taking anticoagulants, even in the absence of overdose. In a study by Soyka et al [50], the authors found that 16% of patients on VKAs had INR values within the therapeutic range.

2-2-3- **Rondu-osler disease**

Hereditary haemorrhagic telangiectasia (HHT) is a rare autosomal dominant disorder characterised by pathological hypertrophy of the blood vessels, leading to the formation of arteriovenous malformations. The exact genetic cause of HHT is attributed to mutations in several genes, including ENG (endoglin), ACVRL1 and SMAD4. These mutations disrupt the normal development and maintenance of blood vessels, leading to the formation of abnormal connections between arteries and veins[51]. Epistaxis in patients with Rendu-Osler disease (ROD) can be attributed to several factors. One factor is the presence of mucocutaneous telangiectasias, which are small arteriovenous malformations most evident on the lips, tongue, oral mucosa, face, chest and fingers [52]. These telangiectasias can lead recurrent bleeding, which is a common manifestation of ROD [53]. Another factor is the development of arteriovenous vessels in the upper gastrointestinal tract, including the stomach and small intestine, which can lead to chronic bleeding and anaemia [54]. In addition, patients with ROD may develop hepatic parenchymal AVMs or vascular shunts, leading to liver cirrhosis and portal hypertension, which can cause bleeding from oesophageal varices [55]. The presence of these AVMs and telangiectasias in various organs may contribute to the occurrence of epistaxis in patients with ROD [56].

2-2-4- Systemic disease

ENT signs are frequently observed in connectivitis, vasculitis and granulomatosis. Epistaxis can be an important diagnostic feature [4].

Vasculitides causing epistaxis include Wegener's diseaseChurg-Strauss syndrome and eosinophilic granulomatosis with polyangiitis. These conditions are associated with inflammation of the blood vessel walls [4].

In Wegener's disease, in addition to epistaxis, the patient may have nasal obstruction and crusty rhinitis [47]. Septal perforation is frequently observed in this condition, triggering recurrent episodes of epistaxis [58].

In the context of connective tissue diseasesatrophic polychondritis may sometimes be implicated in this type of bleeding [59].

Although rare, sarcoidosis can have nasosinus manifestations 1 to 5% of patients. These include nasal crusting, loss of smell, pain and epistaxis [60].

2-3- Essential epistaxis

Fragile vascular staining is the main cause of epistaxis. Peak frequency has been described between the ages of 5 and 20 [61]. Several triggers have been identified, such as scratching, sneezing, intense physical exercise, sun exposure, rhino-logical infections, as well as hormonal variations such as the premenstrual period and pregnancy. Essential epistaxis generally occurs unilaterally and anteriorly. In the literature, several risk factors have been associated with this type of epistaxis, including arterial hypertension, hypercholesterolaemia, smoking, alcohol consumption, use of non-steroidal anti-inflammatory drugs and aspirin, and coagulation disorders [62].

3- DIAGNOSIS OF SEVERITY

The vast majority of cases of epistaxis do not require hospitalisation, with invasive treatment necessary in only 6% of cases [4]. There was still a problem in assessing the severity of epistaxis, which was based subjective criteria. In most studies, epistaxis was classified according to its severity or repetition [63]. In the literature, there is no clear definition of severity, which is often based on subjective criteria such as the estimated volume of bleeding (low, medium or high severity epistaxis), or the location (anterior and/or posterior), with posterior epistaxis being considered as severe or potentially more severe. Some authors [64] believe that when spontaneous epistaxis requires hospitalisation, this may be considered a sign of severity. However, there may also be a bias, as admission may be linked to the frailty of the patient (elderly, comorbid patient) and not just to the epistaxis itself. Nevertheless, hospitalisation implies a degree of clinical instability which may more often than not require invasive treatment, particularly surgery [65]. Thus, in reality, all cases of epistaxis that are subjectively "serious" or "severe" inevitably require hospitalisation. In a study by André et al [66], they classified spontaneous epistaxis as "severe" in cases admission with a previous nasal packing of 48 hours with cessation of epistaxis on D3 of hospitalisation and as "serious" in event of hospitalisation >3 days requiring tamponade at the hospital. double balloon, or in the case of deglobulation with a haemoglobin < 10 g/dl requiring transfusion of packed red blood cells or if invasive surgical treatment and/or selective arterial embolisation under arteriography is required The 2015 SFORL recommendations [4] consider that the severity epistaxis should be assessed on the basis of clinical, haemodynamic and biological criteria:

- An immediate and/or bilateral anteroposterior epistaxis is indicative of severe epistaxis and should be investigated for signs suggestive of hypovolaemic shock.

- Haemorrhagic shock is absolute hypovolaemia secondary to a sudden and significant loss of blood mass, which is also responsible for acute anaemia [67]. (Professional agreement).

The diagnosis of shock is based on the combination of the following signs [68] (level of evidence 4):

- Arterial hypotension (systolic blood pressure <80 mmHg, with pinched differential)

- Tachycardia
- Disturbed consciousness and/or polypnoea and/or cyanosis of the lips and extremities and/or mottling

The risk factors for the severity of severe epistaxis most frequently described in the literature are :

3-1- Age

In most studies, advanced age has been a factor in the severity of epistaxis: in this context, Hadar et al [3] found that age (OR 1.02; CI 1.01-1.023), is significantly correlated with clinical symptoms of epistaxis severity. On the other hand, André et al [66] found no significant differences in terms of severity of epistaxis between patients over 60 and under 60. Paradoxically, the mean age was slightly lower in the severe epistaxis group. Several authors have identified male gender as a factor in the severity of epistaxis: -Hadar et al [3] found that male sex (OR 2.07; CI 1.59-2.69) was significantly correlated with severe clinical symptoms of epistaxis. This predominance of males could be explained by the fact that women impregnated with oestrogen, which protects them more against epistaxis. The role of oestrogen in preventing recurrence of epistaxis was reported by Daniell in 1995 [69]. In a study by André et al [66], they found no significant differences between the groups in terms of sex ratio.

3-3- Season

Several studies have found a higher incidence of admissions due to epistaxis during the winter, probably due to reduced humidity and increased dryness, which can lead to drier mucosa in the nasal cavity and an increased tendency to bleed [9, 70]. In another study, Min et al found that bleeding from the nasal septum generally occurs in winter and spring, when the temperature difference between the inner and outer zones is significant, leading to obvious contraction and relaxation of nasal blood vessels, resulting in dryness of the nasal mucosa and an increased risk of nasal blood vessel rupture. The low temperature and dryness are risk factors for nasal bleeding [38].

3-4- HTA

Most authors consider high blood pressure to be a factor in the severity of epistaxis:-In a meta-analysis [71], the relationship between the severity of epistaxis and hypertension proved controversial. Hypertension was considered to be a risk factor for bleeding, but it was not determined whether it was the cause, as gender and age biases could not be excluded. In another study, Hadar et al [3] found that hypertension (OR 1.76; CI 1.27-2.45) was significantly correlated with severe clinical symptoms of epistaxis.The Multidisciplinary Consensus of the British Rhinological Society only considers arterial hypertension [72] as a risk factor for severe clinical evolution. Consequently, they suggest that this parameter be considered as a major risk factor. However, it should be mentioned that hypertension measured during an episode of epistaxis may not be reliable because it is a stressful event. -A meta-analysis by Jin Min et. Al. 2017 of 10 studies showed an increased odds ratio for epistaxis in patients with hypertension (OR = 1.253; 95% CI: 1.080 - 1.453) [71]. -A 2020 retrospective cohort study by Byun et al demonstrated that hypertension was a significant risk factor for epistaxis with an adjusted hazard ratio of 1.47 (95%

CI: 1.30 - 1.66), they also found that hypertensive patients were more likely to require a posterior nasal dressing [45].

-Another retrospective review by Sethi et. Al. 2017 showed that hypertensive patients presenting to the emergency department were more likely to require a nasal dressing (41.2% versus 30.3%, $p < 0.001$) [73].

-Hayoung et al [74] showed that patients with hypertension were more likely to visit the emergency department for epistaxis and be managed with posterior nasal packing than patients without hypertension. -In a study by André et al [66] severe epistaxis was associated with significantly lower blood pressure and haemoglobinemia. When comparing SAP, DBP and MAP on admission in patients with and without severe epistaxis, no significant difference was found.

3-5- anticoagulants

The role of anticoagulant use in the development of severe epistaxis is controversial from one author to another and from one product to another: Hadar et al [3] found that anti-platelet aggregation or anticoagulation (OR=2.53; IC=1.93-3.33,OR=1.65;IC=1.11-2.44, respectively),were significantly correlated with severe clinical symptoms of epistaxis. -The Multidisciplinary Consensus of the British Rhinological Society considers that anticoagulant treatment carries a higher risk of serious syndrome [72]. -Studies have examined the association between the use of different types of anticoagulant/antiplatelet drugs and the risk epistaxis. The conventional drugs (e.gwarfarin; enoxaparin) were significantly associated with more severe nasal bleeding than new generation oral anticoagulants (e.g. Apixaban Xarelto). [75, 76]. -Tunkel et al consider that although anticoagulants increase the severity and frequency of epistaxis, other preventive and therapeutic measures should first be considered before discontinuing these drugs, unless the bleeding is severe [77]. In this context, nasal saline sprays and nasal emollients are recommended as first-line preventive measures despite the lack of evidence, since they have been shown to significantly improve epistaxis with these moisturising drugs [78, 79].

Unlike previous studies :
Gavin et al did not find that the use of anti-thrombotic drugs was a factor in the severity of epistaxis [80].

-Another study found that the incidence of nosebleeds increased with the increased use of oral anticoagulants, but that the number of patients requiring hospitalisation did not increase [81].

-In a study carried out by André et al [66], they found that the use of drugs altering haemostasis did not appear to be a significant factor in the severity of epistaxis, in contrast to the study by Soyka in which the use of aspirin appeared to be a factor in the severity of epistaxis [50].

3-6- Other co-morbidities

In a study carried out by Chaaban et al, in addition to arterial hypertension, an increase in blood lipid levels, particularly LDL, grade III retinal arteriosclerosis, hyperglycaemia, insufficiency of the arterial blood vessels and the presence of atherosclerosis were observed. cardiac disease and obstructive sleep apnoea/hypopnoea syndrome have been found to be factors in the severity of epistaxis [82]. This can be explained by the alteration of the vascular endothelium by the phenomena of arteriosclerosis responsible for a defect in vascular repair and dragging epistaxis.

3-7- Other

Several other factors responsible for severe forms of epistaxis have been reported in the literature:

-In a retrospective study of 387 patients with epistaxis, Gemechu [83] et al found that blood group O was significantly associated with a severe form of epistaxis O (AOR=3.96, 95% CI = 1.5 to 10.4). The possible reason for the high association observed is that blood group O may be associated with lower expression of Von Willebrand factor, which plays an important role in coagulation, compared with non-O blood groups. As a result, bleeding time is slightly longer in blood group O [84].

Gemechu et al [83] also found that patients who drank coffee daily (OR=2.75, 95% CI=1.0-7.4) and patients who frequently bathed with hot and cold water (OR=4.55, 95% CI=1.1- 18.6) had a greater risk of severe epistaxis.

One of the most common causes of nosebleeds is dry nasal passages, which can be caused by caffeine. This may be because caffeine dries out the body by removing moisture from the mucous membranes of the nasal passages [85].

-In a study carried out in 2022, Andrew et al found that oxygen consumption significantly reduced the risk intervention to stop smoking. epistaxis (OR= 0.45, 95% CI=0.23-0.894; p = 0.028) [86]. Although oxygen is generally associated with nasal dryness when unhumidified, a 2017 systematic review and meta-analysis showed no statistically significant difference in the incidence of epistaxis in patients using unhumidified or humidified low-flow oxygen therapy [71]. Although some causes of epistaxis are known to be very common, sometimes with lightning strikes (due to aneurysmal rupture or post-operative vascular damage), we do not differentiate between epistaxis of local, general or essential origin.

4- THERAPEUTIC MANAGEMENT

4-1- First-line treatment

4-1-1- Assessment of severity and resuscitation procedures

In all patients presenting to the emergency department with epistaxis, the severity of the clinical condition should be assessed initially. In immediately severe cases, resuscitation procedures should be initiated [38,49-52, 87, 88]:

- Oxygen therapy
- Put in two venous approaches,
- Crystalloid infusion,
- Scoop the patient with strict monitoring haemodynamic and respiratory status,
- Biological tests must be taken assess degree of blood spoliation (haemoglobin), the state of haemostasis (PT, APTT, platelets) and to prepare the patient for a possible blood transfusion (Rhesus blood group).
- Transfusion is rare but sometimes compulsory. [89, 90, 91]: (professional agreement): It is suggested that patients be transfused if with acute anaemia, after correction hypovolaemia, from 7 g/dl and from 10 g/dl in patients with acute coronary insufficiency.

These resuscitation procedures must be carried out at the same time as the first steps to stop the bleeding.

4-1-2- Hospitalization

Depending on the severity of the epistaxis and any associated illnesseshospitalisation in a surgical or ENT intensive care unit may be considered. Criteria for hospitalisation include [5, 92] :

- Patients requiring posterior tamponade.

- Patients with anteroposterior tamponade severe diseases such as coronary artery disease, chronic bronchopneumonia, sleep apnoea, immunosuppression, and anaemia with haemoglobin less 9 g/dL.

- When regular follow-up at the consultation is not possible (patients living far from the hospital).

The rate of hospitalisation of emergency department patients for epistaxis varies in the literature from 5% to 17% [66]. In their studies, Varshney et al found that the average length of hospitalisation was 3.2 days (between 1 and 5 days). This period was longer for Chaiyasate et all: 6.2 ± 3.8 days [28].

4-1-3- The first steps to take

The management of epistaxis in adults varies according to whether or not there is bleeding present at the time of the medical consultation. In most cases (around 80%), epistaxis originates in the anterior part of the nose and can be treated locally [94] (professional agreement).Whatever cause of the epistaxis, two steps are standardised:

- Cleaning the nasal cavities: This involves removing blood clots that could be keeping the bleeding going by helping clot to dissolve locally. This can be done by blowing the nose or by suction.

- Prolonged bi-digital compression: Using the thumb and forefinger, compression should be maintained for approximately 10 minutes.

4-1-4- Local haemostasis

If initial measures fail to control epistaxis, local anaesthesia combined with vasoconstriction recommended, unless there are contraindications, before considering diagnostic or therapeutic procedures in cases of prolonged bleeding [95, 96]. This anaesthesia can be achieved using wicks impregnated with 5 and naphazoline (Xylocaine Naphazolinée®), left in place for a maximum of 30 minutes. This combination of local anaesthetic and vasoconstriction is often enough to stop the bleeding, making the examination and subsequent procedures easier. Decisions about the treatment of epistaxis depend on the amount of bleeding, the patient's history and the presence of coagulation disorders. The choice of the type of tamponade to use is influenced by the availability of materials, the amount of bleeding and the patient's overall state of health [97-98].

4-1-4-1-Dabbing

***4-1-4-1-1-* Previous stamping**

Anterior tamponade compresses the anterior three quarters of the nasal cavity. In addition to mechanical pressure, certain materials can have a haemostatic effect [4]. Although there are different types of tamponade No previous tamponade has been shown to be superior. Certain criteria, such efficacy, ease of use, adaptability to the patient and cost, should be taken into consideration when choosing a tamponade [4].Resorbable products include haemostatic wicks such as Surgicel®, synthetic polyurethane sponges (Nasopore®) and haemostatic glues [99]. Contact haemostatics such as Surgicel® and Surgicel Fibrillaire ®, composed of regenerated oxidised cellulose, are present in the form of compresses of different sizes. A small amount of Surgicel ® is applied to the bleeding area in one or two layers. When wet, Surgicel® adheres to the mucosa without impeding breathing, and is then absorbed and eliminated over time [100]. Synthetic polyurethane sponges (Nasopore®) have been shown to be more effective postoperatively than non-absorbable wicks (Merocel®) [101]. Haemostatic adhesives can be used as a first-line treatment for coagulopathy or at the end of surgical procedures [102]. One of these adhesives, Quixil ®, has been compared by Vaiman et al [99] with electric cautery and chemical cautery without finding any difference in terms of bleeding control.

Non-resorbable products include vaseline fatty wicks (Jelonet®), polymeric pads of various lengths (Merocel®, Ultracel®, Netcell®) and calcium alginate wicks (Algosteril®, Urgosorb®). Polymer tampons (Merocel®, Ultracel®, Netcell®) are widely used due to their affordability and effectiveness, but insertion and removal can be uncomfortable [103]. Calcium alginate (Algosteril ®) is less traumatic to remove and reduces the risk of recurrence of epistaxis, allowing the wick to be removed earlier than other types of tamponade [93]. This haemostatic agent, made from algae, is frequently used in neurosurgical and dental procedures and even as a dressing [1].In the case of coagulopathy or anticoagulant or antiplatelet therapy, the French ENT Society recommends the use of absorbable pads to avoid bleeding when the wick is removed [102]. Usually, the duration of a previous tamponade with a non-absorbable material is 48 to 72 hours (SFORL, professional agreement) [102]. Despite its efficacy in stopping anterior bleeding, the risk of recurrence of epistaxis is non-negligible when the tamponade is removed. Some authors have found that 52% of patients with a previous tamponade using a non-absorbable wick had a recurrence of epistaxis when the wick was removed [104]. This rate may be as high as 70% in the presence of a haemostasis disorder [105], and bleeding may even in areas that were previously unaffected due to its traumatic nature [106].

4-1-4-1-2. Posterior tamponade :

In the event of active posterior bleeding or persistent bleeding despite good anterior tamponade, posterior tamponade coupled with anterior tamponade should be used [102]. A 10 cm polymer foam tamponade is usually used for this, although severe posterior epistaxis this method may prove insufficient. In these situations, the use of balloons for posterior tamponade is recommended, with double balloon catheters demonstrating efficacy in 70% of cases. % of cases [107] (level 1 evidence). Despite the lack of approval for the use of Foley catheters, their use remains common due to their effectiveness, availability in emergency departments and affordability, despite the existence of more specific and easier-to-handle catheters. The advantages of these probes include their ease of use, even by non-ENT professionals, and less uncomfortable insertion for the patient. Compared with Foley catheters, double balloon catheters have fewer complications, such as the absence of necrosis of the nasal mucosa [108] (level of evidence 4). The double balloon catheter is generally left in place for 48 to 72 hours, with a recommendation to gradually deflate the balloons after 24 to 48 hours (professional agreement).

4-1-4-1-3- **Antibiotic prophylaxis :**

According to SFORL recommendations, it is not necessary to systematically administer antibiotics when using a nasal swab.

However, their use is recommended if the tampon remains in place for more than 48 hours with a non-absorbable material, or in the presence of other indications requiring antibiotic prophylaxis, such as valvulopathy or immune deficiency. A combination amoxicillin and clavulanic acid should be used during the tampon insertion period and for 5 days after removal. In cases of allergy to penicillin, clarithromycin is recommended (Grade C) [100, 109].

4-1-4-1-4- **Complications:**

The most frequently described complication of mechamation is the recurrence of bleeding during removal, particularly in patients with coagulation disorders. In these situations, the use of absorbable devices is recommended. A recurrence of bleeding when the tampon is removed can Epistaxis can also be caused by removing a tampon too soon. The sensations of stress and pain associated with tampon removal can increase tension, favouring the recurrence of epistaxis. Therefore, prior preparation of the nasal cavity with a non-woven compress impregnated naphazolated xylocaine is recommended before meching, accompanied by the use of a mild analgesic and/or sedative before meching and tampon removal (Professional agreement). Excessive compression and infection can lead to necrosis of the nasal mucosa. This necrosis can cause adhesions between the septum and the lateral wall, and more rarely septal perforations. Suffering of the mucosa is often due to excessive compression, especially with over-inflated balloon devices or when water rather than air is used to inflate the pads. The risk of mucosal damage increases with the use of bilateral tampons and their repetition, favouring the development of adhesions and septal perforations. To reduce the risk of necrosis, it is advisable to deflate the balloon every 6 . The catheter should be kept in place for a maximum of 72 hours, and it is recommended that the balloons are gradually deflated after 24 to 48 hours (Professional agreement).

Particular attention must be paid to the areas of contact between the probe and the skin to avoid nasal eschar formation.

4-1-4-2. Cauterisation: There are several methods of cauterisation:

- Chemical cauterisation using silver ball or stick form is considered less aggressive for the mucosa than the use of chromic or trichloroacetic acid. According to the professional agreement, this method should only be used on the vascular stain [94]. The application of the stick involves firm pressure on the bleeding site for 5 to 10 seconds [94, 110].

- Electrical cauterisation is performed using a single or bipolar electrode, in accordance with the recommendations of the professional agreement [111]. It can be applied to the vascular spot or to an angiomatous area in the inferior turbinate without the need for tamponade [4].

- The possibility of septal perforation after bilateral cauterisation remains controversial. Some practitioners perform bilateral chemical cauterisation without observing perforation [112] (level of evidence 3).

However, it has not been established that bilateral electrocoagulation is without risk of complications, which is why caution is recommended when performing it at the same time (professional agreement). Several authors advocate cauterisation of an identified bleeding site as the optimal management of epistaxis in adults, allowing both anterior and posterior epistaxis to be controlled [94, 110].

A study by Suprya et al [113] demonstrated that 100% of patients with anterior epistaxis and 64% of patients with posterior epistaxis were successfully managed by cautery (bipolar or silver nitrate). In another study, Soyka et all [114] found that 84% of epistaxis was stopped by cautery; the failure rate was higher with chemical than electrical cautery (22% versus 12%). Some authors have found that electrical cautery is more effective than chemical cautery in the acute phase of bleeding [110].

4-1-4-3- Other local treatments :

Various therapeutic approaches are described in the medical literature for the treatment of epistaxis. Among these, humidification of the nasal cavity by nasal instillation of saline water is recommended to prevent the formation of scabs [115]. The application oils or ointments to protect the mucosa and prevent it drying out is also suggested. mild and recurrent epistaxis in children, the use an intranasal antiseptic cream has been considered as an alternative to silver nitrate cauterisation [116]. A single-blind randomised controlled trial compared an antiseptic cream containing 0.5% neomycin and 0.1% chlorhexidine (Naseptine) with a placebo in children aged between 1 and 16 years. The results showed a 26% reduction in the absolute risk of recurrent epistaxis in the month following treatment [117].

- In addition, the use of nasal antiseptic creams, including compounds such as oxytetracycline hydrochloride and polymyxin B sulphate, has demonstrated similar efficacy to cauterisation alone in the treatment of recurrent epistaxis

[118, 119].

4-2- Second-line management: regional haemostasis :

Surgical treatment options and embolisation are generally considered as a second line of treatment for epistaxis [102]. They considered when bleeding persists despite adequate initial treatment, or if the epistaxis relapses after removal of the strands.

4-2-1- Embolisation :

The first embolisation was performed by Sokoloff in 1974[120]. Before considering embolisation to epistaxis, it is essential to diagnostic angiography. This step is crucial in guiding treatment by identifying the cause and location of the bleeding. It also allows us to check the anterograde flow of the ophthalmic arteries, rule out any occlusion of the carotid artery and assess any anatomical variants or risky anastomoses during embolisation in the territory of the external carotid arteries [27].
Embolisation may target various arteries, including the sphenopalatine artery, the maxillary artery, the external carotid artery or the ethmoidal arteries. Technical success has been estimated at between 80 and 88% [121], with complications occurring in 8 to 13% of cases. Technical improvements, the expertise of operators, and developments in embolisation materials and agents explain the improvement in results over time [122-125].

The most commonly described complications of embolisation are haemorrhagic recurrence, facial neuralgia, septal perforation, rhinosinusitis and otitis media. Although rare, more serious complications have been described, such as cerebrovascular accidents (CVA) or occlusion of the central retinal artery, with percentages varying between 0 and 2% depending on the series [126]. In a large series by Brinjikji et all [127] involving 64,289 patients, comparing arterial ligation and embolisation for epistaxis, the author revealed a significantly higher rate of stroke after embolisation compared with arterial ligation (0.9% [41 out of 4440] vs 0.1%...).[34/64 289], p <0,0001).

4-2-2- Arterial ligation :

Arterial ligation, which is less frequently used nowadays, may be necessary in the absence of suitable equipment or staff trained to perform embolisation. Ligation may involve different arteries, such as the sphenopalatine artery, the maxillary artery, the anterior and posterior ethmoidal arteries, or even the external carotid artery [128]. To ligate the sphenopalatine artery, after locating the posterior-superior fontanel, a vertical incision is made in the mucosa and periosteum, approximately 1 cm anterior to the tail of the middle turbinate. A mucosal flap then removed as far as the sphenopalatine foramen, and the artery and periosteum are located. Ligation is performed using clips or bipolar coagulation. This technique is indicated for persistent posterior epistaxis or in cases of surgical injury to this artery. The success rate is up to 95% [129, 130]. Ligation of the maxillary artery is done endoscopically, after performing a wide meatotomy, the median two-thirds of the posterior prey of the maxillary sinus is milled. The maxillary artery can be located and ligated.In cases of recurrent high epistaxis, the anterior and posterior ethmoidal arteries may be ligated. A cutaneous incision starting at the root of the eyebrow and extending para lateronasally to the periosteum allows access to these arteries in order to ligate them. However, this method presents a risk of optic nerve damage [131]. Although the literature shows variable results, arterial ligation is associated complications such as persistent crusting (up to 33% in some series), nasal dryness and persistent posterior discharge [123], sometimes with paresthesia of the palate and nasal cavity [132]. In a comparison of embolisation and arterial ligation, although embolisation was found to be more effective than arterial ligation (94% vs 89%) [133], there was no difference in the risk of mortality or blindness between the two methods. However, embolisation was significantly more expensive.

4-3- Therapeutic indications

A treatment approach for epistaxis based on the model developed by Dufour and colleagues [134] (level of evidence 4) has been developed:

❖ **Benign epistaxis**: Bleeding is not very profuse, often unilateral and intermittent, with no general repercussions. Bleeding is usually localized at the level of the vascular spot during anterior rhinoscopy.

- If there has been previous bleeding, an initial bidigital manual compression should always be applied for a few minutes.

So ineffective :
- Anterior licking with haemostatic wicks.
- Endoscopic electrocoagulation under local anaesthetic if a previous lesion is visible.

If unsuccessful :
- Anteroposterior tamponade with double balloon probe
In the event persistent failure :

- Consideration of posterior epistaxis as refractory, requiring more advanced endovascular treatments:

- Coagulation or embolisation of the sphenopalatine artery.
- If this fails, ligation of the anterior ethmoidal artery.

❖ **Severe epistaxis from the outset:** heavy bleeding, often bilateral with anterior and posterior bleeding. Possibly severe in terms of its abundance or recurrence, requiring hospitalisation:

General actions :

- Management of possible haemorrhagic shock.
- Placement of two venous lines and infusion of macromolecules.
- Transfusion of compatible blood if necessary.
- Rest and administration anxiolytics to reduce stress-related hypertensive flare-ups.

- General treatment to haemostasis: Dicynone (3 amp. IM/d).

Local actions :

- Initial anterior tamponade.
- Follow-up of the treatment regimen for less severe forms if necessary (Figure 1).

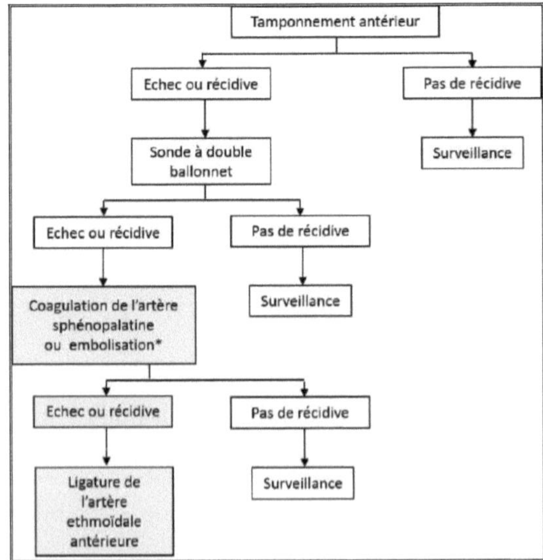

Figure 1: Treatment algorithm for epistaxis developed by Dufour et all [134].

4-4- Special form: Patient on anticoagulant (AC) or antiplatelet agent (AAP)

In patients on anticoagulant (AC) or antiplatelet (AAP) therapy, the management of epistaxis requires a tailored approach:

❖ **For patients on anticoagulants:**

- In the first instance, the use of resorbable devices such as Surgicel® or Nasopore® is preferred.

- In the event of persistence, tamponade with non-absorbable devices (Merocel® or Algosteril®) or a greasy wick may be considered.

- If the bleeding persists, especially if the epistaxis has a posterior component, the delicate placement of a double balloon catheter may be considered.

- Severe forms epistaxis require hospitalisation.

- Continuation of treatment with AC or PAA depends on the effectiveness of buffering and the risk of thrombosis, provided there is no overdose.

- For severe or recurrent epistaxis, specialist advice (haematologists and/or cardiologists) is required to adapt the treatment.

❖ **For patients on PAAs:**

- return to haemostasis depends on the type antiplatelet agent used, sometimes taking up to 10 days.

- Discontinuation of the PAA may be considered in the event recurrent epistaxis, taking into account the risk of thrombosis.

- In the case of aspirin treatment, the efficacy nor the risk of haemorrhage is dose-dependent between 75 and 300 mg/day. [135]

- In the case of dual therapy (aspirin + clopidogrel), a temporary pause in clopidogrel may be considered, with the advice a cardiologist to assess the risks and benefits.

- The same considerations apply to the new P2Y12 inhibitors, Efient® (prasugrel) and Brilique® (ticagrelor), which are associated with an increased risk of epistaxis.

- In the event of uncontrolled bleeding, platelet transfusion is recommended, requiring varying amounts depending on the drug: 5 units for patients on aspirin compared with at least 10 units for clopidogrel or prasugrel. In the case of ticagrelor, even a massive transfusion of platelet packed red blood cells has not been shown to be effective [136] (level 4 evidence).

❖ **For patients on VKA :**

- Any epistaxis in a patient on VKA requires careful monitoring of the INR.

- The return to coagulation stopping VKAs varies from 2 to 5 days without taking vitamin K.

- In emergency situations, prothrombin complex concentrate (PCC or PPSB) rapidly restores the anticoagulant effect at a dose of 25 units/kg.

- The dose of vitamin K depends on the degree of overdose and the state of the liver, enabling the synthesis of coagulation factors to be accelerated within 8 hours.

- Management is determined by regular biological monitoring, in line with HAS recommendations for severe haemorrhagic cases, the criteria for which are in line with those for severe epistaxis. This information is presented in Figures 2 and 3.

INR mesuré	Mesures correctrices recommandées en fonction de l'INR mesuré et de l'INR cible INR cible 2,5 (fenêtre entre 2 et 3)	 INR cible ≥ 3 (fenêtre 2,5 - 3,5 ou 3 -4,5)
INR < 4	• Pas de saut de prise • Pas d'apport de vitamine K	
4 ≤ INR < 6	• Saut d'une prise • Pas d'apport de vitamine K	• Pas de saut de prise • Pas d'apport de vitamine K
6 ≤ INR < 10	• Arrêt du traitement • 1 à 2 mg de vitamine K par voie orale (1/2 à 1 ampoule buvable forme pédiatrique) (grade A)	• Saut d'une prise • Un avis spécialisé est recommandé (ex. cardiologue en cas de prothèse valvulaire mécanique) pour discuter un traitement éventuel par 1 à 2 mg de vitamine K par voie orale (1/2 à 1 ampoule buvable forme pédiatrique)
INR ≥ 10	• Arrêt du traitement • 5 mg de vitamine K par voie orale (1/2 ampoule buvable forme adulte) (grade A)	• Un avis spécialisé sans délai ou une hospitalisation est recommandé

Figure 2: Correction of INR in a patient on VKA [137].

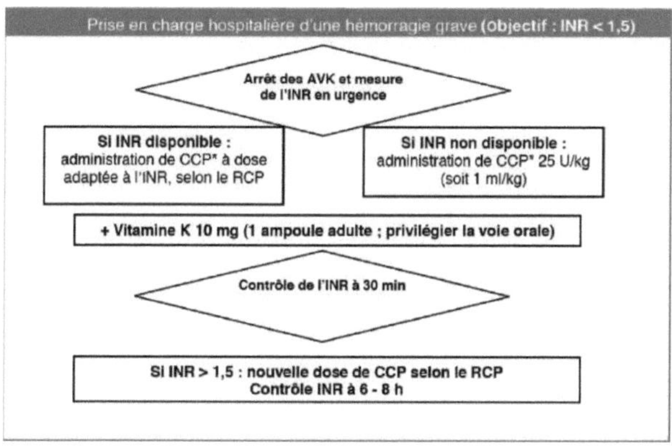

Figure 3: Correction of INR in a patient on VKA serious bleeding [137] (professional agreement)

Discontinuation of VKA anticoagulation is possible without relay in patients with a low risk of thrombosis and who have been treated with non-absorbable material which to be removed after 48 to 72 hours with the least risk. recurrence of epistaxis. The therapeutic window without VKAs will therefore be reduced to 48 - 72 hours. In patients at high risk of thrombosis who have had to stop taking VKAs, a relay course of LMWH should be started once the bleeding is under control. dose of VKA reintroduction depends on whether the epistaxis occurred within the therapeutic INR range or in the context of an overdose. The VKA should be reintroduced in hospital, under clinical and biological supervision [137] (professional agreement).

❖ **Patients on oral anticoagulants**

Management of Direct Oral Anticoagulants (DAA) in the event serious haemorrhage or emergency surgery: For patients with a low thromboembolic risk: AODs can be discontinued after specialist cardiological advice, without a repeat treatment. Normalisation of coagulation should be achieved within 24 to 72 hours, taking into account the type of AOD, its dose and the patient's renal function.For patients presenting a high thromboembolic risk: discontinuation of AODs should be followed by heparin [138] (professional consensus). In the event of serious haemorrhage or urgent surgery, only patients on Pradaxa® (dabigatran) can have an antidote (Praxbind®) at a dose of 5 mg intravenously over 5 to 10 minutes. Anti-Xa molecules (Xarelto®, Eliquis®, Lixiana®) do not currently have an antidote [139].

5- EVOLUTION: RISK FACTORS FOR RECURRENCE OF EPISTAXIS

5-1-Age

In addition to the risk of severity, several authors have identified advanced age as a factor in the recurrence of epistaxis: In a series of 4120 patients, Chaaban et al revealed by multivariate analysis that age> 75 years was an independent predictor of readmission for epistaxis [82]. In another study, Addisson et al [140] found that increasing age > 70 years was a factor in recurrence of epistaxis (p=0.042; OR=1.71, CI=1.02- 2.85).

5-2- Gender

In addition to the risk of severity, male gender has been identified by several authors as a factor in the recurrence of epistaxis:-Kallenbach et al found that male gender was an independent predictor of subsequent readmission due to recurrent epistaxis (OR = 1.756; CI = 1.155-2.668) [141]. - -For Khan et al, the recurrence rate was 13.9%, higher men [142]. -In another study, Chaaban et al revealed by multivariate analysis that male gender was an independent predictor of readmission [82].

5-3- HTA

The risk of epistaxis recurrence due to hypertension has been studied by several authors: Abrich et al conducted a retrospective cohort study of over 50 potential risk factors for spontaneous recurrent epistaxis and showed that hypertension may increase the risk of epistaxis recurrence by inducing arteriosclerotic changes in the nasal vessels [143]. In another study Jackson et al examined the factors associated with active and refractory epistaxis. They showed that arterial hypertension was a frequent factor in the recurrence of epistaxis [144]. On the contrary, other studies have found that there was no significant difference in recurrence between hypertensive and non-hypertensive patients [74].

5-4- anticoagulants

Anti-thrombotic treatment has been shown to cause recurrent and heavier bleeding and an increase in incidence of blood transfusions [72]. In addition, numerous studies have shown that the use of anticoagulants results in longer hospitalisation due to recurrence of epistaxis [72, 142].Also in this context, Kallenbach et al found that taking oral anticoagulants was an independent predictor of subsequent readmission due to recurrent epistaxis (OR = 1.731; CI = 1.046-2.865). [141]. Similarly, Adisson et al [140] found that taking oral anticoagulants was a factor in recurrence of epistaxis ($p<0.0001$, OR=4.94, CI=3.06- 9.16) independent of other factors.In a study of 444 patients, Stanković et al found that patients on acetyl salicylic acid had more frequent recurrences than the general population (1.83 ± 0.47 vs 1.2 ± 0.3; $p = 0.002$) [145].

Jackson et al also showed that association of arterial hypertension and aspirin intake were factors in active and refractory epistaxis. [144]. In contrast to these studies, Goljo et al [146] and Sauter et al [147] found that the use of anticoagulants was associated with a shorter hospital stay for epistaxis.

5-5- Other co-morbidities

Numerous studies have found no correlation between recurrent epistaxis and cardiovascular comorbidity [105, 148]. However, Abrich et al found that diabetes mellitus in association with arterial hypertension are factors in the recurrence of epistaxis due to alteration of the vascular endothelium [143]. Using multivariate analysis, Chaaban et al revealed that diabetes is an independent predictor of readmission for epistaxis [82].

5-6- Site of bleeding and nature of treatment

In a 2014 study, Ando et al found that factors for epistaxis recurrence were unidentified bleeding points, the treatment strategy used during initial bleeding episode, and posterior nasal bleeding [105]. Similarly, So Jeong et al found posterior epistaxis and anterior packing alone were factors in the recurrence of epistaxis [148].

In the same context, Adisson et al [140] found that failure to identify the site of bleeding ($p=0.008$; OR=4.84, CI=2.91-8.92) and posterior packing ($p<0.0001$; OR=5.23, CI=3.52- 10.97) were factors in the recurrence of epistaxis.

In a study by Yuji et al [149], an unidentified bleeding site was predictive of an increased risk of recurrent epistaxis (OR=5.67, 95% CI= 1.83-17.55, $p=0.003$) and electrocautery was predictive of a decreased risk of recurrent epistaxis (OR= 0.07, 95% CI= 0.03- 0.17, $p= 0.0001$). The rate recurrent epistaxis was significantly lower in patients who underwent electrocautery as initial treatment compared with those who did not (6.4% versus 40.7%, $p<0.01$), and was significantly higher in those who underwent tamponade compared with those who did not (39.5% versus 15.9%, $p<0.01$). In another study, Shargorodsky et al found that treatment with electrical or chemical cautery increased the success rate and reduced the risk of recurrent bleeding [150].

5-7- Other

-Kallenbach et al found that hereditary haemorrhagic telangiectasia was an independent predictor of subsequent readmission due recurrent epistaxis (OR = 13.216; 95% CI=5-34) [141]. - -Chaaban et al revealed by multivariate analysis that obstructive sleep apnoea syndrome was an independent predictor of readmission for epistaxis. [82].

-Based on a multivariate analysis in a case series of 653 patients, Cohen et al [93] found that patients treated with nasal surgery and having anaemia had an independent risk of early readmission for epistaxis.

-Jackson et al examined the factors associated active and refractory epistaxis. They showed that alcohol abuse and that septal deviation, spurring and mucosal abnormality were anatomical factors in having such nasal cavity bleeding [144].

6- LIMITS OF THE STUDY

Although this study has enabled us to highlight the factors of severity and recurrence of epistaxis, it does have certain shortcomings: The population studied is small compared with those observed in the literature, which will affect the power of the results found. A sampling error should be noted, since we excluded cases of common epistaxis and patients who were not hospitalised, which reduced the number of non-severe forms of epistaxis (which represented only 80% of all cases). cases epistaxis), making the comparison between two groups unrepresentative.We not have information on the outcome of all patients discharge from hospital. In this case, the number of recurrences of epistaxis is underestimated. Epistaxis is one of the most frequent emergencies in otorhinolaryngology (ENT). It is usually trivial, but can be serious and life-threatening. This severity may be due to its abundance or repetition. Several factors can influence the severity of epistaxis, including the patient's condition, the aetiology and the nature of the treatment. The clinician an important role to play in identifying "dangerous forms of initial or secondary epistaxis and initiating early, comprehensive and effective management in order to improve the prognosis.

REFERENCES

1. Walker TW, Macfarlane TV, McGarry GW. The epidemiology and chronobiology of epistaxis: an investigation of Scottish hospital admissions 1995-2004. Clin Otolaryngol 2007; 32:361-365.

2. Timsit CA, Bouchène K, Olfatpour B, Tsigaridis P, Herman P, Tran Ba Huy P. Epidemiology and clinical findings in 20,563 patients attending the Lariboisière Hospital ENT Adult Emergency Clinic. Ann Otolaryngol Chir Cervicofac 2001; 118:215-24.

3. Hadar A, Shaul Ch, Ghantous J, Tarnovsky Y, Cohen A, Zini A. Risk Factors for Severe Clinical Course in Epistaxis Patients. Ear, Nose & Throat Journal 2023 :1-6.

4. Epistaxis 2015 Report of the French ENT Society. 2015.

5. Pollice PA, Yoder MG. Epistaxis: a retrospective review of hospitalized patients. Otolaryngol Head Neck Surg 1997; 117:49-53.

6. Ari K, Collins R. Outpatient Management of Epistaxis During COVID-19 to Reduce Inpatient Stay: A Quality Improvement Project. Cureus. Oct 2022;14(10):e30858.

7. Parajuli R. Evaluation of Etiology and Treatment Methods for Epistaxis: A Review at a Tertiary Care Hospital in Central Nepal. Int J Otolaryngol. 2015;2015:283854.

8. Li HY, Luo T, Li L, Liu Y, Zhai X, Wang XD. Etiology and clinical characteristics of primary epistaxis. Ann Transl Med. 31 Jan 2023;11(2):96.

9. Ahn EJ, Min HJ. Age-specific associations between environmental factors and epistaxis. Front Public Health. 2022;10:966461.

10. ElAlfy MS, Tantawy AAG, Eldin BEMB, Mekawy MA, Mohammad YA

elAziz, Ebeid FSE. Epistaxis in a Pediatric Outpatient Clinic: Could It be an Alarming Sign? Int Arch Otorhinolaryngol. 3 June 2021;26(2):e183 90.

11. Althaus AE, Lüske J, Arendt U, Dörks M, Freitag MH, Hoffmann F, et al. Treating epistaxis - who cares for a bleeding nose? A secondary data analysis of primary and secondary care. BMC Fam Pract. 15 Apr 2021;22(1):75.

12. Purkey MR, Seeskin Z, Chandra R. Seasonal variation and predictors of epistaxis. The Laryngoscope. Sep 2014;124(9):2028 33.

13. Tabassom A, Dahlstrom JJ. Epistaxis. In: StatPearls [Internet]. Treasure Island (FL): StatPearls Publishing; 2023 [cited 3 Oct 2023]. Available from: http://www.ncbi.nlm.nih.gov/books/NBK435997/

14. Kemal O, Sen E. Does the weather really affect epistaxis? B-ENT. 2014;10(3):199 202.

15. Myszkowska D, Bazgier M, Brońska S, Nowak K, Ożga J, Woźniak A, et al. Scraping nasal cytology in the diagnostics of rhinitis and the comorbidities. Sci Rep. August 25, 2022;12(1):14492.

16. Ruggiero R, Motta G, Massaro G, Rafaniello C, Della Corte A, De Angelis A, et al. Pharmacological, Technological, and Digital Innovative Aspects in Rhinology. Front Allergy. 15 Dec 2021;2:732909.

17. Cingoz F, Oz BS, Arslan G, Guler A, Sahin MA, Gunay C, et al. Is chronic obstructive pulmonary disease a risk factor for epistaxis after coronary artery bypass graft surgery? Cardiovasc J Afr. 2014;25(6):279 81.

18. Douglas CM, Tikka T, Broadbent B, Calder N, Montgomery J. Patterns of hospital admission in 54 501 patients with epistaxis over a 20-year period in Scotland, UK. Clin Otolaryngol Off J ENT-UK Off J Neth Soc Oto-Rhino-Laryngol Cervico-Facial Surg. dec 2018;43(6):1465 70.

19. Bermüller C, Bender M, Brögger C, Petereit F, Schulz M. [Epistaxis and

anticoagulation - a medical and economic challenge?]. Laryngorhinootologie. Apr 2014;93(4):249 55.

20. Langsted A, Nordestgaard BG. Smoking is Associated with Increased Risk of Major Bleeding: A Prospective Cohort Study. Thromb Haemost. Jan 2019;119(1):39 47.

21. Harrison-Woolrych M, Härmark L, Tan M, Maggo S, van Grootheest K. Epistaxis and other haemorrhagic events associated with the smoking cessation medicine varenicline: a case series from two national pharmacovigilance centres. Eur J Clin Pharmacol. Jul 2012;68(7):1065 72.

22. Soyka MB, Schrepfer T, Holzmann D. Blood markers of alcohol use in epistaxis patients. Eur Arch Oto-Rhino-Laryngol Off J Eur Fed Oto-Rhino-Laryngol Soc EUFOS Affil Ger Soc Oto-Rhino-Laryngol - Head Neck Surg. August 2012;269(8):1917 22.

23. McGarry GW, Gatehouse S, Hinnie J. Relation between alcohol and nose bleeds. BMJ. 10 Sep 1994;309(6955):640.

24. McGarry GW, Gatehouse S, Vernham G. Idiopathic epistaxis, haemostasis and alcohol. Clin Otolaryngol Allied Sci. Apr 1995;20(2):174 7.

25. Gilyoma JM, Chalya PL. Etiological profile and treatment outcome of epistaxis at a tertiary care hospital in Northwestern Tanzania: a prospective review of 104 cases. BMC Ear Nose Throat Disord. 5 Dec 2011;11(1):8.

26. Varshney S, Saxena RK. Epistaxis: A retrospective clinical study. Indian J Otolaryngol Head Neck Surg Off Publ Assoc Otolaryngol India. 2005;57(2):125 9.

27. Krajina A, Chrobok V. Radiological diagnosis and management of epistaxis. Cardiovasc Intervent Radiol. Feb 2014;37(1):26 36.

28. Chaiyasate S, Roongrotwattanasiri K, Fooanan S, Sumitsawan Y. Epistaxis

in Chiang Mai University Hospital. J Med Assoc Thai. 2005;88(9):1282 6.

29. Hern JD, Coley SC, Hollis LJ, Jayaraj SM. Delayed massive epistaxis due to traumatic intracavernous carotid artery pseudoaneurysm. J Laryngol Otol. Apr 1998;112(4):396 8.

30. Karkanevatos A, Karkos PD, Karagama YG, Foy P. Massive recurrent epistaxis from non-traumatic bilateral intracavernous carotid artery aneurysms. Eur Arch Otorhinolaryngol. 9 Jul 2005;262(7):546 9.

31. Béquignon E, Teissier N, Gauthier A, Brugel L, De Kermadec H, Coste A, et al. Emergency Department care of childhood epistaxis. Emerg Med J EMJ. August 2017;34(8):543 8.

32. Jégoux F, Métreau A, Louvel G, Bedfert C. Paranasal sinus cancer. Eur Ann Otorhinolaryngol Head Neck Dis. Dec 2013;130(6):327 35.

33. Shovlin CL. Supermodels and disease: insights from the HHT mice. J Clin Invest [Internet]. 15 Nov 1999 [cited 30 Nov 2017];104(10):1335 6. Available from: http://www.jci.org/articles/view/8730

34. Vi CHUM. Epistaxis in emergencies: 140 cases Cone-beam imaging: ENT applications Management of epistaxis: a case report. Epistaxis in patients with Rendu Osler disease by nasal spraying of bevacizumab Sternberg canal . 2011;28.

35. Lund VJ, Stammberger H, Nicolai P, Castelnuovo P, Beal T, Beham A, et al. European position paper on endoscopic management of tumours of the nose, paranasal sinuses and skull base. Rhinol Suppl. 2010;22:1 143.

36. Chandler JR, Goulding R, Moskowitz L, Quencer RM. Nasopharyngeal angiofibromas: staging and management. Ann Otol Rhinol Laryngol. 29 July 1984;93(4 Pt 1):322 9.

37. Sarhan NA, Algamal AM. Relationship between epistaxis and hypertension:

A cause and effect or coincidence? J Saudi Heart Assoc. Apr 2015;27(2):79 84.

38. Min HJ, Kang H, Choi GJ, Kim KS. Association between Hypertension and Epistaxis: Systematic Review and Meta-analysis. Otolaryngol Neck Surg. 1 Dec 2017;157(6):921 7.

39. Zampaglione B, Pascale C, Marchisio M, Cavallo-Perin P. Hypertensive Urgencies and Emergencies. Hypertension. Jan 1996;27(1):144 7.

40. B, Yavuz B, Yildiz E, Ozkan S, Ayturk M, Sen O, et al. A possible cause of epistaxis: Increased masked hypertension prevalence in patients with epistaxis. Braz J Otorhinolaryngol. 2015;(xx):1 5.

41. Terakura M, Fujisaki R, Suda T, Sagawa T, Sakamoto T. Relationship between blood pressure and persistent epistaxis at the emergency department: a retrospective study. J Am Soc Hypertens JASH. Jul 2012;6(4):291 5.

42. Kikidis D, Tsioufis K, Papanikolaou V, Zerva K, Hantzakos A. Is epistaxis associated with arterial hypertension? A systematic review of the literature. Eur Arch Oto-Rhino-Laryngol Off J Eur Fed Oto-Rhino-Laryngol Soc EUFOS Affil Ger Soc Oto-Rhino-Laryngol - Head Neck Surg. Feb 2014;271(2):237 43.

43. Bereda G. Hypertensive Urgency and Anterior Epistaxis Caused by Antihypertensive Medication Noncompliance: A Case Report. Open Access Emerg Med OAEM. 3 Feb 2023;15:47 51.

44. Recht M, Chitlur M, Lam D, Sarnaik S, Rajpurkar M, Cooper DL, et al. Epistaxis as a Common Presenting Symptom of Glanzmann's Thrombasthenia, a Rare Qualitative Platelet Disorder: Illustrative Case Examples. Case Rep Emerg Med. 2017;2017:8796425.

45. Byun H, Chung JH, Lee SH, Ryu J, Kim C, Shin JH. Association of Hypertension With the Risk and Severity of Epistaxis. JAMA Otolaryngol--Head Neck Surg. Jan 2021;147(1):1 7.

46. Bibbins-Domingo K, U.S. Preventive Services Task . Aspirin Use for the Primary Prevention of Cardiovascular Disease and Colorectal Cancer: U.S. Preventive Services Task Force Recommendation Statement. Ann Intern Med. June 21, 2016;164(12):836 45.

47. Shehab N, Sperling LS, Kegler SR, Budnitz DS. National Estimates of Emergency Department Visits for Hemorrhage-Related Adverse Events From Clopidogrel Plus Aspirin and From Warfarin. Arch Intern Med. 22 Nov 2010;170(21):1926 33.

48. Rainsbury JW, Molony NC. Clopidogrel versus low-dose aspirin as risk factors for epistaxis. Clin Otolaryngol Off J ENT-UK Off J Neth Soc Oto-Rhino-Laryngol Cervico-Facial Surg. June 2009;34(3):232 5.

49. Watson MG, Shenoi PM. Drug-induced epistaxis? J R Soc Med. March 1990;83(3):162 4.

50. Soyka MB, Holzmann D, Probst R. New developments in epistaxis. 2013;290 2

51. Andorfer KEC, Seebauer CT, Dienemann C, Marcrum SC, Fischer R, Bohr C, et al. HHT-Related Epistaxis and Pregnancy-A Retrospective Survey and Recommendations for Management from an Otorhinolaryngology Perspective. J Clin Med. 13 Apr 2022;11(8):2178.

52. Macri A, Wilson AM, Shafaat O, Sharma S. Osler-Weber-Rendu Disease. In: StatPearls [Internet]. Treasure Island (FL): StatPearls Publishing; 2023 [cited 3 Oct 2023]. Available from: http://www.ncbi.nlm.nih.gov/books/NBK482361/

53. Ramanandafy H, Andriamahenina FPP, Tiaray MH, Nandimbiniaina AM, Razafindrasoa AZ, Razafimpihanina S, et al. Pulmonary arteriovenous malformation revealing Osler-Weber-Rendu disease: A case report. Clin Case Rep. 17 Jan 2022;10(1):e05294.

54. Mahfoudhi M, Khamassi K. Rendu-Osler disease: a diagnosis not to be ignored. Pan Afr Med J. 17 Sep 2015;22:40.

55. Litsou E, Basiari L, Tsirves G, Psychogios GV. Hereditary Hemorrhagic Telangiectasia With Multiple Ear, Nose, and Throat (ENT) Manifestations: A Case Report. Cureus. 15(7):e42706.

56. Chin CJ, Rotenberg BW, Witterick IJ. Epistaxis in hereditary hemorrhagic telangiectasia: an evidence based review of surgical management. J Otolaryngol - Head Neck Surg. 12 Jan 2016;45:3.

57. Tunkel DE, Anne S, Payne SC, Ishman SL, Rosenfeld RM, Abramson PJ, et al. Clinical Practice Guideline: Nosebleed (Epistaxis). Otolaryngol--Head Neck Surg Off J Am Acad Otolaryngol-Head Neck Surg. Jan 2020;162(1_suppl):S1 38.

58. Diamantopoulos II, Jones NS. The investigation of nasal septal perforations and ulcers. J Laryngol Otol. July 2001;115(7):541 4.

59. Cardenas-Garcia J, Farmakiotis D, Baldovino B-P, Kim P. Wegener's granulomatosis in a middle-aged woman presenting with dyspnea, rash, hemoptysis and recurrent eye complaints: a case report. J Med Case Reports. 3 Oct 2012;6:335.

60. Kirsten A-M, Watz H, Kirsten D. Sarcoidosis with involvement of the paranasal sinuses - a retrospective analysis of 12 biopsy-proven cases. BMC Pulm Med. 26 Dec 2013;13(1):59.

61. Anatomique R. Treatment of epistaxis. 2010;

62. Reyre A, Michel J, Santini L, Dessi P, Vidal V, Bartoli J-M, et al. Epistaxis: The role of arterial embolization. Diagn Interv Imaging [Internet]. 1 Jul 2015 [cited 30 Jun 2018];96(7 8):757 73. Available from: https://www.sciencedirect.com/science/article/pii/S2211568415002132?vi

a%3Dihub.

63. Biet A, Liabeuf S, Strunski V, Fournier A. Serious spontaneous epistaxis and hypertension in hospitalized patients. Eur Arch Otorhinolaryngol 2011; 268:1749-53.

64. Page C, Biet A, Liabeuf S, Strunski V, Fournier A. Serious spontaneous epis-taxis and hypertension in hospitalized patients. Eur Arch Otorhinolaryngol 2011;268:1749-53.

65. Klossek JM, Dufour X, de Montreuil CB, et al. Epistaxis and its management: an observational pilot study carried out in 23 hospital centres in France. Rhinology 2006;44:151-5.

66. André N, Klopp-Dutote N , Biet-Hornstein A, Strunski V ,Page C. Cardiovascular risk and severity factors in patients admitted to hospital for spontaneous epistaxis. European Annals of Otorhinolaryngology, Head and Neck diseases 2018; 135: 119-122.

67. Riou B., Vivien B., Langeron O. Choc hémorragique traumatique. Les Essentiels 2005, p. 457-474.

68. Shakeel M, Trinidade A, Iddamalgoda T, Supriya M, Ah-See KW. Routine clotting screen has no role in the management of epistaxis: reiterating the point. Eur Arch Otorhinolaryngol 2010 Oct;267(10):1641-4.

69. Daniell HW. Estrogen prevention of recurrent epistaxis. Arch Otolaryngol Head Neck Surg 1995;121:354.

70. Fletcher LM. Epistaxis. Surgery (Oxford). 2009;27(12):512-517.

71. Min HJ, Kang H, Choi GJ, Kim KS. Association between Hypertension and Epistaxis: Systematic Review and Meta-analysis. Otolaryngol Head Neck Surg 2017;157(6):921-927.

72. INTEGRATE (The National ENT Trainee Research Network). The British Rhinological Society multidisciplinary consensus recommendations on the hospital management of epistaxis. J Laryngol Otol 2017;131:1142-1156.

73. Sethi RKV, Kozin ED, Abt NB, Bergmark R, Gray ST. Treatment disparities in the management of epistaxis in United States emergency departments. Laryngoscope 2017;128(2):356-362.

74. Hayoung B, Jae Ho Ch, Seung H, Jiin R, Changsun K, Jeong-Hun Sh. Association of Hypertension With the Risk and Severity of Epistaxis. JAMA Otolaryngol Head Neck Surg 2021;147(1):34-40.

75. Yaniv D, Zavdy O, Sapir E, Levi L, Soudry E. The Impact of Traditional Anticoagulants, Novel Anticoagulants, and Antiplatelets on Epistaxis. Laryngoscope 2021;131(9):1946-1951.

76. Buchberger AMS, Baumann A, Johnson F, et al. The role of oral anticoagulants in epistaxis. Eur Arch Otorhinolaryngol 2018; 275(8): 2035-2043.

77. Tunkel DE, Anne S, Payne SC, et al. Clinical Practice Guideline: Nosebleed (Epistaxis). Otolaryngol Head Neck Surg. 2020;162(1_suppl):S1- S38.

78. Loughran S, Spinou E, Clement WA, Cathcart R, Kubba H, Geddes NK. A prospective, single-blind, randomized controlled trial of petroleum jelly/Vaseline for recurrent paediatric epistaxis. Clin Otolaryngol Allied Sci 2004;29(3):266-269.

79. Wen Z, Wang W, Zhang H, Wu C, Ding J, Shen M. Is humidified better than non-humidified low-flow oxygen therapy? A systematic review and meta-analysis. J Adv Nurs 2017;73(11):2522-2533.

80. Gavin D, Kwee YG, Puneet T, Sangeeta M, Bhaskar R, Raghav CD. Anti thrombotics and their impact on inpatient epistaxis management: a tertiary

centre experience. Irish Journal of Medical Science 2022; 191:1621-1629.

81. Althaus AE, Arendt U, Hoffmann F, et al. Epistaxis and anticoagulation therapy: an analysis based on health insurance data from Lower Saxony. HNO 2021;69:206-12. Erratum in: HNO 2021;69:98..

82. Chaaban MR, Zhang D, Resto V, et al. Factors influencing recurrent emergency department visits for epistaxis in the elderly. Auris Nasus Larynx 2018;45:760-4.

83. Gemechu A, Gelila B, Hayat M, Abebayehu Ch, Melese M, Mohammed H et al. Epistaxis and Its Associated Factors Among Precollege Students in Southern Ethiopia. Journal of Blood Medicine 2021:12 1-8.

84. Adhikari P, Pramanik T, Pokharel R, Khanal S. Relationship between blood group and epistaxis among Nepalese. Nepal Med College J. 2008;10(4):264-265.

85. Nowak D, Jasionowski A. Analysis of the consumption of caffeinated energy drinks among Polish adolescents Int. J Environ Res Public Health 2015;12:7910-7921.

86. Andrew R, Steven E, Rebecca M, Samba B. Risk Factors and Management for Epistaxis in a Hospitalized Adult Sample. SMRJ. 2022;7(2).

87. Le Tulzo Y. Diagnosis of shock. Réanimation. Emergency medicine M3. Year 2012-2013

88. Shakeel M, Trinidade A, Iddamalgoda T, Supriya M, Ah-See KW. Routine clotting screen has no role in the management of epistaxis: reiterating the point. Eur Arch Otorhinolaryngol. 2010 Oct;267(10):1641-4

89. Huet O., Harrois A., Duranteau J. Transfusion sanguine en réanimation. Congrès national d'anesthésie et de réanimation 2008. Les Essentiels, p. 467-480.© 2008 Elsevier Masson SAS. All rights reserved.

90. Professional recommendations. Management of antivitamin K overdose, bleeding risk situations and haemorrhagic events in patients treated with antivitamins K in hospital and outpatient settings - HAS - Service de bonnes pratiques professionnelles - April 2008

91. Carson JL, Carless PA, Hebert PC, transfusion threshold an other strategies for guiding allogeneic red blood cell transfusion. Cochrane database syt rev 2012

92. Barnes ML, Spielmann PM, White PS. Epistaxis: a contemporary evidence based approach. Otolaryngol Clin North Am. Oct 2012;45(5):1005 17.

93. Cohen O, Shoffel-Havakuk H, Warman M, Tzelnick S, Haimovich Y, Kohlberg GD, et al. Early and Late Recurrent Epistaxis Admissions: Patterns Incidence and Risk Factors. Otolaryngol-Head Neck Surg. Sep 2, 2017;157(3):424 31.

94. Pope, L.E. and C.G. Hobbs, Epistaxis: an update on current management. Postgrad Med J, 2005. 81(955): p. 309-14.

95. McGarry, G., Nosebleeds in children. Clin Evid, 2006(15): p. 496-9.

96. Chiu TW, McGarry GW. Prospective clinical study of bleeding sites in idiopathic adult posterior epistaxis. Otolaryngol Head Neck Surg. 2007 Sep;137(3):390-3.

97. Badran K, Malik TH, Belloso A. Randomized controlled trial comparing Merocel and RapidRhino packing in the management of anterior epistaxis. Clin Otolaryngol. 2005; 30(4) : 333-7.

98. Singer AJ, Blanda M, Cronin K. Comparison of nasal swabs for the treatment of epistaxis in the emergency department: a randomized controlled trial. Ann Emerg Med. 2005; 45 (2): 134-9.

99. Cohn B. Are prophylactic antibiotics necessary for anterior nasal packing in

epistaxis? Ann Emerg Med 2015;65:109 11.

100. Pepper C, Lo S, Toma A. Prospective study of the risk of not using prophylactic antibiotics in nasal packing for epistaxis. J Laryngol Otol. 2012;126:257 9.

101. D'Arbonneau-Rolland V. Accidents hémorragiques sous antagonistes de la vitamine K chez la personne âgée : à propos de 86 cas. *Thèse de Docteur en médecine]. Nancy: Université Henri Poincaré; 2002. Available at: http://docnum.univ-lorraine.fr.basesdoc. univ-lorraine.fr/prive/SCDMED_T_2002_D_ARBONNEAU_ROLLAND_VIRGINI E.pdf?

102. Duranteau J. New SFAR recommendations in haemorrhagic shock. Transfus Clin Biol 2015;22:188.

103. Chaaban MR, Zhang D, Resto V, Goodwin JS. Demographic, Seasonal, and Geographic Differences in Emergency Department Visits for Epistaxis. Otolaryngol-Head Neck Surg 2017;156:81 6.

104. Côrte FC, Orfao T, Dias CC, Moura CP, Santos M. Risk factors for the occurrence of epistaxis: Prospective study. Auris Nasus Larynx [Internet] 2017 [cited 2018 March 3]; Available from: http://linkinghub.elsevier.com/retrieve/pii/S0385814617300950

105. Ando Y, Iimura J, Arai S, Arai C, Komori M, Tsuyumu M, et al. Risk factors for recurrent epistaxis: importance of initial treatment. Auris Nasus Larynx 2014;41:41 5.

106. Nguyen-Khac É, Gournay N, Tiry C, Thevenot T, Skaf C-É, Leroy M-H. Portable hemoglobinometer for bedside monitoring of capillary blood hemoglobin in patients with acute gastrointestinal hemorrhage. Presse Médicale. August 2006;35:1131 7.

107. McClurg SW, Carrau R. Endoscopic management of posterior epistaxis: a review. Acta Otorhinolaryngol Ital. 2014, Feb;34(1):1-8.

108. Civelek B, Kargi AE, Sensoz O, Erdogan B. Rare complication of nasal packing: alar region necrosis. Otolaryngol Head Neck Surg. 2000, Nov;123(5):656-7.

109. Gungor H, Ayik MF, Gul I, Yildiz S, Vuran O, Ertugay S, Kanyilmaz H, Erturk U. Infective endocarditis and spondylodiscitis due to posterior nasal packing in a patient with a bioprosthetic aortic valve. Cardiovasc J Afr. 2012, Mar 12;23-2.

110. Spielmann PM, Barnes ML, White PS. Controversies in the specialist management of adult epistaxis: an evidence-based review. Clin Otolaryngol Off J ENT-UK Off J Neth Soc Oto-Rhino-Laryngol Cervico- Facial Surg. oct 2012;37(5):382 9.

111. Frikart, L. and A. Agrifoglio, Endoscopic treatment of posterior epistaxis. Rhinology, 1998. 36(2): p. 59-61.

112. Felek SA1, Celik H, Islam A, Demirci M, Bilateral simultaneous nasal septal cauterization in children with recurrent epistaxis. Int J Pediatr Otorhinolaryngol. 2009 Oct;73(10):1390-3.

113. Supriya M, Shakeel M, Veitch D, Ah-See KW. Epistaxis: prospective evaluation of bleeding site and its impact on patient outcome. J Laryngol Otol. 20 Jul 2010;124(7):744 9.

114. Soyka MB, Rufibach K, Huber A, Holzmann D. Is severe epistaxis associated with acetylsalicylic acid intake? The Laryngoscope. Jan 2010;120(1):200 7.

115. Wurman LH, Sack JG, Flannery J V, Lipsman RA. The management of epistaxis. Am J Otolaryngol. 13(4):193 209.

116. Nichols A, Jassar P. Paediatric epistaxis: diagnosis and management. Int J Clin Pract. August 2013;67(8):702 5.

117. Kubba H, MacAndie C, Botma M, Robison J, O'Donnell M, Robertson G, et al. A prospective, single-blind, randomized controlled trial of antiseptic cream for recurrent epistaxis in childhood. Clin Otolaryngol Allied Sci. Dec 2001;26(6):465 8.

118. Ozmen S, Ozmen OA. Is local ointment or cauterization more effective in childhood recurrent epistaxis. Int J Pediatr Otorhinolaryngol. June 2012;76(6):783 6.

119. Ruddy J, Proops DW, Pearman K, Ruddy H. Management of epistaxis in children. Int J Pediatr Otorhinolaryngol. Apr 1991;21(2):139 42.

120. Srinivasan V, Patel H, John DG, Worsley A. Warfarin and epistaxis: should warfarin always be discontinued? Clin Otolaryngol Allied Sci. Dec 1997;22(6):542 4.

121. Christensen NP, Smith DS, Barnwell SL, Wax MK. Arterial embolization in the management of posterior epistaxis. Otolaryngol--Head Neck Surg Off J Am Acad Otolaryngol-Head Neck Surg. Nov 2005;133(5):748 53.

122. Andersen PJ, Kjeldsen AD, Nepper-Rasmussen J. Selective embolization in the treatment of intractable epistaxis. Acta Otolaryngol (Stockh). March 2005;125(3):293 7.

123. Fukutsuji K, Nishiike S, Aihara T, Uno M, Harada T, Gyoten M, et al. Superselective angiographic embolization for intractable epistaxis. Acta Otolaryngol (Stockh). May 8, 2008;128(5):556 60.

124. Sadri M, Midwinter K, Ahmed A, Parker A. Assessment of safety and efficacy of arterial embolisation in the management of intractable epistaxis. Eur Arch Oto-Rhino-Laryngol Off J Eur Fed Oto-Rhino- Laryngol Soc EUFOS Affil

Ger Soc Oto-Rhino-Laryngol - Head Neck Surg. 21 June 2006;263(6):560 6.

125. Strach K, Schröck A, Wilhelm K, Greschus S, Tschampa H, Möhlenbruch M, et al. Endovascular treatment of epistaxis: indications, management, and outcome. Cardiovasc Intervent Radiol. 7 Dec 2011;34(6):1190 8.

126. Mames RN, Snady-McCoy L, Guy J. Central retinal and posterior ciliary artery occlusion after particle embolization of the external carotid artery system. Ophthalmology. Apr 1991;98(4):527 31.

127. Brinjikji W, Kallmes DF, Cloft HJ. Trends in Epistaxis Embolization in the United States: A Study of the Nationwide Inpatient Sample 2003- 2010. J Vasc Interv Radiol. Jul 2013;24(7):969 73.

128. Meaudre E, Bordes J, Prunet B, Cathelinaud O, Kenane N, Palmier B, Goutorbe P. Massive haemorrhage during craniofacial trauma. traite'e par ligature de la carotide externe ; Annales Françaises d'Anesthésie et de Réanimation 2008 ;27 :252-255.

129. Voegels RL, Thomé TC, Vasquez Iturralde PP, Butugan O. Endoscopic ligation of the sphenopalatine artery for severe posterior epistaxis. Otolaryngol Head Neck Surg 2001;124:464-7.

130. Snyderman CH, Carrau RI. Endoscopic ligation of the sphenopalatine artery for epistaxis; Operative techniques in otolaryngology--head and neck surgery 1997;8(2):85-89.

131. Viehweg TL, Roberson LB, Hudson JW. Epistaxis: Diagnosis and Treatment. American Association of Oral and Maxillofacial Surgeons J Oral Maxillofac Surg 2006;64:511-518.

132. Snyderman CH, Goldman SA, Carrau RL, Ferguson BJ, Grandis JR. Endoscopic sphenopalatine artery ligation is an effective method of treatment for posterior epistaxis. Am J Rhinol. Apr 1999;13(2):137 40.

133. Strong EB, Bell DA, Johnson LP, Jacobs JM. Intractable epistaxis: transantral ligation vs. embolization: efficacy review and cost analysis. Otolaryngol--Head Neck Surg Off J Am Acad Otolaryngol-Head Neck Surg. Dec 1995;113(6):674 8.

134. Dufour X, Lebreton JP, Gohler C, Ferrié JC, Klossek JM: Epistaxis. In: Encycl Méd Chir Oto-rhino-laryngologie Elsevier Paris SAS; 2010: 1-7 [Article 20-310-A-10].

135. Baigent & al. Collaborative metaanalysis of randomized trials of antiplatelets therapy for prevention of death, myocardial infarction, and stroke in high risks patients. BMJ 2002 324;71-86.

136. Platelet transfusion: products, indications Method Recommendations for clinical practice, HAS recommendation, October 2015.

137. Management of antivitamin K overdose, bleeding risk situations and haemorrhagic events in patients treated with antivitamins K in outpatient and hospital settings April 2008 (SYNTHESE DES RECOMMANDATIONS PROFESSIONNELLES, HAS GEHT).

138. Anticoagulants in France in 2014: , summary and monitoring, ANSM 2014

139. Pernod et Al, Prise en charge des complications hémorragiques graves et de la chirurgie, niveau de preuve en urgence chez les patients recevant un anticoagulant 2013 Annales françaises d'anesthésie et de réanimation

140. Addison A, Paul C, Kuo R, Lamyman A, Martinez-Devesa P, Hettige R. Recurrent epistaxis: predicting risk of 30-day readmission, derivation and validation of RHINO-ooze score. Rhinology 2017; 55: 99-105.

141. Kallenbach M, DittbernerA, Boeger D, Buentzel J, Kaftan H, Hoffmann K et al. Hospitalization for epistaxis: a population based healthcare research study in Thuringia, Germany. European Archives of Oto-Rhino-Laryngology 2020;

277:1659-1666. -

142. Khan M, Conroy K, Ubayasiri K. Initial assessment in the management of adult epistaxis: systematic review. J Laryngol Otol 2017; 131:1035-1055.

143. Abrich V, Brozek A, Boyle TR, et al. Risk factors for recurrent spontaneous epistaxis. Mayo Clin Proc 2014;89(12):1636-1643.

144. Jackson KR, Jackson RT. Factors associated with active, refractory epistaxis. Arch Otolaryngol Head Neck Surg 1988;114:862-5.

145. Stanković P, Hoch S, Rudhart S, Stojković S, Wilhelm T. The pattern of epistaxis recurrence in patients taking prophylactic acetylsalicylic acid (ASA) from a 10 year cohort. European Archives of Oto-Rhino-Laryngology 2023; 280:1723-1730.

146. Goljo E, Dang R, Iloreta A, Govindaraj S. Cost of management in epistaxis admission: impact of patient and hospital characteristics. Laryngoscope 2015; 125(12):2642-7.

147. Sauter TC, Hegazy K, Hautz WE. Epistaxis in anticoagulated patients: fewer hospital admissions and shorter hospital stays on rivaroxaban compared to phenprocoumon. Clin Otolaryngol 2018; 43:103-108.

148. So Jeong K, So Jeong L, Yu Jin G, Sohl P, Jung Ho B. Characteristics and Risk Factors of Recurrent Epistaxis in Geriatric Patients. Korean J Otorhinolaryngol-Head Neck Surg 2021;64(8):548-53.

149. Yuji A, Jiro I, Satoshi A, Chiaki A, Manabu K, Matsusato T. Risk factors for recurrent epistaxis: Importance of initial treatment. Auris Nasus Larynx 2014; 41: 41-45.

150. Shargorodsky J, Bleier BS, Holbrook EH. Outcomes analysis in epistaxis management: development of a therapeutic algorithm. Otolaryngol Head Neck Surg 2013; 149:390-398.

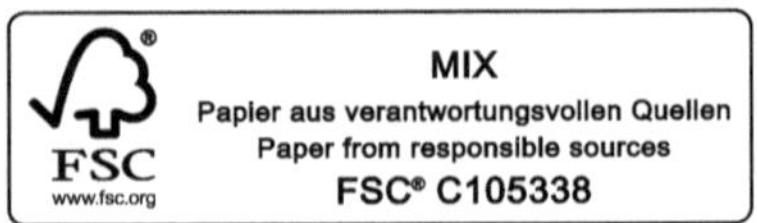

Printed by Books on Demand GmbH, Norderstedt / Germany